Table of Contents

INTRODUTION

Whether it's just a temporary thing or a permanent habit, juicing is growing in popularity, especially among health-conscious people. Points need to be considered carefully, I recommend juicing to all family and house hold to practice and it has a great benefit to human health. Get all the information you need here.

JUCING YOUR WEIGHT OUT

CHAPTER ONE

START SUPPLYING YOUR LIFE WITH JUICE

Juice can be integrated into the everyday way of life to improve sound living and it is likewise a decent way on expanding the day to day admission of fruit and vegetable.

THE PRIMARY

However, for most people, making juice is a chore and a hassle, or however, it is a welcome alternative for those who enjoy juice highly recommended as it's better to go in person than buy the juice product.

All juice products must be treated and processed to ensure these homemade juices are preferred due to their integrity and shelf life close.

However, when making homemade juices, it's important to remember that it's important to consume the juice product as soon as it's ready. Exposed air effectively loses much of its advertised initial value.

Also, juices are consumed regularly; Getting into the habit of limiting your juices to fresh fruit is not optimal.

The idea that many fruits are naturally high in sugar and not Very high in fiber, causing negative buildup of sugar liver body system. This can lead to diabetes and weight gain problems.

A better alternative is complementary fruits and Vegetables come together to form a savory concoction that's both delicious and good health. Plus healthy fats and lean protein Diet is one of the benefits.

CHAPTER TWO

BENEFIT OF JUICE TO ONES HEALTH

As more and more people indulge in this form of healthy eating, Consuming fruits and vegetables is becoming more and more popular Juice it instead of eating it whole shape.

However, while scientists and nutritionists are divided as to the benefits of eating these products whole versus sipping juice, there is still no proven data to justify or support either option.

ADVANTAGES OF JUICE

However, some prior knowledge is required before actually making juice-drink and enduring characteristic of an individual Lifestyle.

Juice is one way to get all the fruit, according to research.

Herbal requirements to effectively body systems, although there is no active addition of fiber. It's definitely a more effective way to get nutrients into your body's system without putting too much pressure on your digestive system to break down fiber.

For those who dislike eating fruits and vegetables, juice may be a more acceptable alternative.

There are also various repetitions for juicing Brew more comfortable and even tastier. Juice combo is good to include in your sourcing of vegetable and fruit recipes exercise.

Most juice recipes contain fruit parts that would be wasted in traditional consumption methods.

However, when making juice, pits, skins, seeds, and other parts are included in the process because they are known to contain rich sources of important nutrients that are typically systematically discarded.

Processed juices usually require some sort of heating process to extend the shelf life of the product, and this tends to kill the enzymes. And with juicing, it can be avoided and the enzymes will still remain intact without been damage.

CHAPTER THREE

SOLID JUICE RECIPES

Finally, there are many positive reasons encouraging more people to start drinking juice. These include the opportunity to save money as you can buy fruit in bulk. Eating plan increases a person's energy and vitality levels.

Below is a unit a number of the foremost well-liked juice recipes for avid juicers.

Lemon Apple - a pair of apples, 1 lemon, one in. slice of ginger. Because of its high content of flavonoids, it is a healthy remedy for colds. It conjointly contains a contemporary, zesty flavor that's terribly tonic.

Plain O'O.J - four medium oranges. Remember to incorporate it as much white membrane as attainable is additionally a decent plan here Rich in bioflavonoids. But during this case it might be higher Avoid the thought the thought a full peel because it will add sourness. And raw style, creating the juice quite unpleasant taste.

Alkaline juice - one cup spinach, 1/2 cup cucumber, 2 stems

Celery with leaves. Three carrots and 1/2 apple. The skin of dark inexperienced cucumbers give a supply of chlorophyll, this is a photochemical that helps build red blood cells.

 Cucumbers conjointly contain silicon oxide, a kind of mineral Good for skin.

Berry pastiche - a pair of cups strawberries, 2 cups blueberries and one and a half cups of raspberries. Berries area unit well-liked

It breaks down quickly and simply, creating it excellent for juicing.

It's a straightforward flushing action. As a wonderful supply of antioxidants, Anthocyanins, flavonoids, and ellagic acid all have glorious anti-cancer and anti-cardiac effects.

Pomegranate juice - five pomegranates. For this formula, use solely the seeds and discard the remainder of the fruit. However, the seeds area unit troublesome to grind, therefore you'll retrieve ends up in a liquidizer.

CHAPTER FOUR

JUICE OUT FAT

Incorporating juice-drinking exercise into your weight loss diet arranges could be terribly effective thanks to turn. , it ought to be noted that the juicing method ought to ideally embody each vegetables and fruits.

Burn out the fat with juice

Juice is also a good ingredient for any detoxic exercise. It can be used as a meal replacement or when a fasting plan is included position.

If the juice is meant to detoxic, it works Eliminates toxins and fats that have accumulated over time in the body system.

These juices act as cleansers that make them an ideal alternative to heavy, unhealthy meals. Drinking juices can also be a healthier and more viable way to lose weight.

Most juice recipes designed for weight loss are very good nutritious and satisfying to ensure that individuals do not have to be hunger, resort to supplementing it with other foods. It also usually contains ingredients that are part of a particular product.

A combination of toxin-scavenging properties fat it's also a good idea to ensure that all ingredients used in juice recipes are fresh ingredients and that everything is thoroughly washed before actually making the juice.

Below is some iteration to help you on your quest to skim the fat;

Chokeberry Fiber - Apples are an excellent cleanser and berries provide mineral supplements.

Green Pineapple - This concoction is refreshing, delicious and extremely filling.

Orange Pineapple Chili; Rich in vitamin C and enzymes that can break down mucus buildup in the body and also boosts metabolism.

Ginger Pear - A wonderful laxative and good for digestion.

CHAPTER FIVE

JUICE FOR THE KIDS

In such cases, both parents and children often have a hard time when come to addressing the problem of consumption of the vegetables and fruits provided meal. However, it has been found to solve this problem in most cases eradicated or at least reduced to manageable levels.

For the kids

Juices are a great and fun way to nourish a growing child's body and ensure optimal development of the body.

Technology has designed a mixture that is pleasant to drink and, above all, has a refreshing effect after an intense gaming session. There is something to do.

However, it is recommended to dilute the juice for younger children, as the concentrated form may be too much for the undeveloped body.

Teenagers and older children should have a hard time drinking concentrated juices. The introduction of juicing for children should be a gradual process with early stages of dilution. Choosing delicious fruit is much better and less likely to be rejected by your child. It's also a good idea to start by choosing individual juices before moving on to combinations. This allows your child's body systems and taste buds to get used to the introduction into a healthy daily eating plan.

Changing the juice and adding variety is definitely an attractive feature for children, who will be captivated by the colors and flavors, reflected in the variety.

Once your favorite juices have been identified, serve them as often as possible

It is possible and beneficial without boring the child. Use Favorites Based on juice, sometimes a small amount can be added

Other fruits and vegetables to further improve the nutritional content of the juice. Some popular options are apple juice, pineapple, and carrots juice, orange juice, grape juice.

CHAPTER SIX

JUICE FOR ANTI AGING

Juicing is not the new fad for combating the natural aging process. While it makes sense to choose this healthier and cheaper method, it is no less effective at starving the aging process.

LOOKING YOUNGER WITH JUICE

Juices offer a combination of everything, thus benefiting the body vital vitamins, minerals, amino acids, essential fatty acids.

These fruits and vegetables are usually used for juice Full of anti-aging and life-sustaining elements; therefore, it is decided to incorporate regular juice practice benefit greatly.

Antioxidants and substances that neutralize free radicals this system ideally offers excellent anti-aging potential service.

Eating a diet rich in vitamins and minerals is a key factor in fighting the aging process, and one of the most enjoyable ways to do this is with juice.

Colorful fruits and vegetables are especially useful for anti-aging. Fruits such as oranges, cherries, tangerines, apples, blueberries, cranberries, melons, bananas, grapes, berries, kiwis and mangoes are all known for their anti-aging properties.

These can be taken in combination or individually depending on what you have. Suitable for individual tastes.

Speaking of vegetables which are Carrots, pumpkin, red kale, broccoli and spinach are abundant and equally beneficial for anti-aging.

Apple and Carrot Detoxic – 1 apple, 1 slice of ginger, 1 carrot, ½ cup or water. Its excellent properties create healthy skin and eliminate it Removing toxins from the body is why this juice is so popular a lot.

Cholesterol Burner – 1 apple, 1/2 cucumber, 4 celery stalks, 1/2 cup water. This juice also helps to properly regulate high cholesterol levels in the body and fight stomach upsets along with its more obvious anti-aging properties.

CHAPTER SEVEN

JUICE HELP IN DETOXIFICATION

The juicing process is ideal for detoxifying the body system as it improves the absorption of enzymes, vitamins and minerals that greatly benefit the immune system.

DETOXIFICATION

Juicing nutrient-rich organic vegetables and fruits coats the cells in the body with alkaline juices released from these juice preparations, releasing acids and removing toxins through various elimination channels in the body. It is useful to Parts of the body that play an important role in filtering such toxins include the lungs, kidneys, skin, and other functions such as urination and defecation.

The enzymes released by these juices also help in the digestive process, where proteins break food down into nutrients. This is an important feature as most adults have exhausted their natural digestive enzymes by the age of 30.

Therefore, the external help provided by the juice is definitely beneficial to the digestive process, as it is essential to the detoxification regiment the body naturally requires.

These added juices cleanse the body and carry the right amount of oxygen and nutrients straight through, because when the body is riddled with toxins, it cannot absorb the nutrients available in its natural intake of normal foods. Helps break down toxins for... cells and tissues.

Some of the ideal ingredients for the juicing process Detoxic includes lettuce, dark green kale, carrots and beets, leafy greens, coriander, parsley, celery, collards, endive, spinach, dandelion leaves, both purple and green cabbage, Lemon.

Some People Practicing This Detoxic Regiment Regularly testify that cravings for sweets have disappeared food and they can eat regularly and healthily without it Fight it probably because the body can do it works best with a detoxification session.

CHAPTER EIGHT

SOCIAL SHOWCASING

It has already been established that drinking juice is very healthy exercise training. This is one of the ensuring factors an individual's likelihood of developing a medical problem is greatly reduced by reducing the risk of disease

The Juice Drinking Habit Is Proven to Be a Habit Everyone Should Consider its benefits.

BEING HEALTHY

There are some very specific combinations that can be used on a regular basis to produce the ideal effect on the body system, thereby resisting the development of all conceivable diseases.

One of these is drinking a beetroot combo that is said to significantly reduce the risk of heart disease, stroke, Alzheimer's disease and dementia.

Bright red juice contains chemical nitrates that dramatically lower blood pressure in nearly everyone taking this compound.

Another juice combination is with pomegranate content, which is important for reducing cardiovascular risk, but this should be done with caution due to its very high potassium content. It is also said to help relieve heart disease and reduce the symptoms of diabetes. Another benefit of consuming tomato juice is resistance to developing chronic diseases such as cancer and coronary artery disease. This is avoided due to the high content of a carotenoid called lycopene in tomatoes.

Foods that can be used to fight disease, or at least reduce the risk of disease, include broccoli, Brussels sprouts, butternut squash, collards, Chinese broccoli, kale, spinach, parsley, collards, mustard greens, chard, beets, carrots, Cauliflower, cucumber, pepper, sweet potato, lettuce, celery.

The regular combination of these juices helps maintain the chemical balance of the body's systems, allowing the body to function at its highest level and effectively prevent disease.

CHAPTER NINE

JUICE HELP IN STRESS RELIEVE

Almost all adults and children experience a series of stresses at various points in their daily lives. In most cases this is acceptable to the point of no longer possible. When this happens, it almost always affects your health.

RELIEVE STRESS

Fruit and vegetable juices have long been best-known to cut back stress and restful properties. Please take the time to seem into this it's undoubtedly price Taking Healthy Alternatives rather than Taking Medications to alleviate Stress effort.

While the ingredients in apples, cherries, and blueberries area unit best-known health-promoting ingredients, flavonoids improve respiratory organ operate, and during this optimum respiration position, the best quantity of Oxygen circulates well, reducing the interior pressure that builds up within the body. Relax you'll feel high levels of stress and this ultimately helps cut back your stress levels.

These ingredients additionally facilitate relax the arteries; reduce the danger of ordinarily caused disorder Emphasis.

Banana, strawberry and peppermint smoothie Lemon will facilitate cut back stress and provides you AN overall feeling of relaxation bodily sensation the advantages of the higher than ingredients area unit as a result of once catecholamine levels rise, the body desires additional water-soluble vitamin and this can't be naturally elicited by the figure, thus it should be replenished from external sources.

Bananas contribute stress-relieving properties, peppermint that contains application, incorporates a cooling result on the body, et al aid digestion, making AN overall result that combats the presence of great stress.

New findings show that regular consumption of fruits and vegetables in the form of juices can provide significant benefits to the body's systems.

CONCLUSION

Drinking juice is not as healthy as eating whole fruits and vegetables.

When juicing, the juice is obtained from fresh fruits and vegetables. The liquid contains most of the vitamins, minerals and phytochemicals (phytonutrients) found in fruit. But whole fruits and vegetables also contain healthy fiber, most of which is lost during juicing.

Juices help reduce cancer risk, boost the immune system, remove toxins from the body, aid digestion, and help you lose weight.

However, there is no scientific evidence that extracted juices are healthier than the juices obtained by eating the fruits and vegetables themselves.